THE PHYSICIAN IN
ENGLISH HISTORY

Linacre Lecture, 1913
St John's College, Cambridge

THE PHYSICIAN IN ENGLISH HISTORY

by

NORMAN MOORE, M.D.

Fellow of the Royal College of Physicians
Honorary Fellow of St Catharine's College
Consulting Physician to St Bartholomew's Hospital

Cambridge
at the University Press
1913

CAMBRIDGE UNIVERSITY PRESS
Cambridge, New York, Melbourne, Madrid, Cape Town,
Singapore, São Paulo, Delhi, Mexico City

Cambridge University Press
The Edinburgh Building, Cambridge CB2 8RU, UK

Published in the United States of America by Cambridge University Press, New York

www.cambridge.org
Information on this title: www.cambridge.org/9781107615861

First published 1913
First paperback edition 2013

A catalogue record for this publication is available from the British Library

ISBN 978-1-107-61586-1 Paperback

THE PHYSICIAN IN ENGLISH HISTORY

The first physician mentioned in English history is Cynifrid, who appears in the *Historia Ecclesiastica Gentis Anglorum* of Bede. The passage in which his name occurs and in which his very words are quoted deserves consideration. He was present at the death of Etheldreda abbess of Ely and at her disinterment sixteen years later. He used to tell that when ill she had a great swelling under the jaw. "They bid me," he said, "to cut that swelling so that the hurtful humour which was therein might flow out. When I did it she seemed for two days somewhat better, so that many thought that she might recover from her weakness. But on the third day she was attacked by her former pains, and being snatched from the world changed pain and death for everlasting health and life." He goes on to describe the uncovering of the saint's body sixteen years later. She lay as if asleep. The bystanders "pointed out to me the wound of the incision, which I had made, cured ; so that in a wonderful way instead of an open and gaping wound with which she was buried there appeared very slender traces of a scar." Had we been present we should probably have thought that the incision had thoroughly drained the abscess and that the edges of the wound had fallen together. What was the nature of the swelling ? A remark which immediately follows Cynifrid's description shows that the swelling was not an incident of an acute disease but had existed for some time in the saint's neck. "She was much delighted with this kind of illness and used to say ' I know truly that I ought to bear the weight of disease in my neck in which I mind me that in my girlhood I used to carry the useless burden of necklaces, and I believe that therefore Providence wills that I should suffer pain in my neck that thus I may be cleared from the accusation of vanity when now for gold and pearls the redness and heat of a swelling stand out in my neck.'" These are the words and meditations of a patient who has long had a suppurating swelling in the neck and such a swelling is rarely other than tuberculous. The words "ac solita dicere" exclude the sudden onset and rapid course of an attack of bubonic plague. Cynifrid, who witnessed the illness, does not say a word of other deaths. The hymn writer who points out how his subject differs from those of Virgil and of Homer

> Bella Maro resonet, nos pacis dona canamus ;
> Munera nos Christi, bella Maro resonet.
> Carmina casta mihi, fedæ non raptus Helenæ ;
> Luxus erit lubricis, carmina casta mihi.

does not utter a word of prevalent plague or of the deaths at Ely of contemporary nuns.

"There are some," says Bede earlier in this chapter of his fourth book, "who say that by the spirit of prophecy she both foretold the pestilence of which she was to die and openly made known to all present the number of those who from her monastery should be carried from the world by it."

The Saxon Chronicle states that Etheldreda died in 679 but mentions no epidemic of plague at Ely in that year. Thus there is no real evidence that Etheldreda died, as has been conjectured, of the plague, while the actual account of her illness and the evidence of an eyewitness Cynifrid as to it establishes the strong probability that she died of tuberculosis. Cynifrid, the first mentioned of English physicians, whose opinion on a patient is thus set forth in Bede, was not a monk for he stood outside hearing the brethren and sisters singing within and the distinct voice of the newly elected abbess Sexberg suddenly calling out

Sit gloria nomini Domini

and was after that asked to come into the choir to see the disentombed body of abbess Etheldreda. Nor is there any mention of his being in holy orders.

We must not apply the ideas of our own day in which every man is educated and examined into his profession to the days of the Heptarchy. Cynifrid had probably read medicine and he practised it with sufficient success to give his patients confidence in him, for he had been attached to the abbey of Ely for more than sixteen years.

The latest new book on medicine of his time was that contained in the Liber Etymologiarum of Isidore of Sevile.

If Cynifrid had read this treatise he knew the

name of Hippocrates, son of Asclepius, born in the island of Cos, who is the only physician mentioned in the book on medicine, and except Varro the only author. He would have divided diseases into acute, chronic and superficial and could have given some definition of sixteen acute, and thirty-eight chronic diseases and of twenty-one diseases which are seen on the surface of the skin. Guided by Isidore, Cynifrid would have placed Etheldreda's disease under the heading Parotida and it is easy to imagine him after feeling the surface of the tumour expressing himself in Saxon to the abbess in the words of Isidore

Parotide sunt duritie vel collectiones que ex febribus aut ex aliquo alio nascuntur in aurium vicinitate : unde et parotide sunt appellate.

As regards treatment Cynifrid would have explained that there were three kinds of cure : by diet and regimen, by drugs and by cutting

with an iron instrument, and would have re-
commended the last. He felt the fluid inside
the tumour and the appearances described later
show that he made his incision in a part likely
to drain the whole. He had never dissected
the human body and such knowledge of Anatomy
as he had may have been derived from the
eleventh book of Isidore, a lengthy and confused
account of the external appearances and internal
organs of the body, without a single paragraph
of precise description. He knew from this the
lines of Ovid on man's erect posture

> Pronaque cum spectent animalia cetera terram,
> Os homini sublime dedit : cælumque tueri
> Jussit, et erectos ad sidera tollere vultus.

I can recall their quotation, in the course of
his teaching, by a lecturer on Anatomy whose
remarks in every other particular differed from
those of Isidore, so capable of everlasting use
are the phrases of poets.

If Cynifrid had looked into the rest of the Liber Etymologiarum his mind contained a large collection of information from many branches of knowledge. He had met with the names and some of the words of Virgil, Horace, Cicero, Lucretius, Lucilius, Ennius, Plautus, Terence, Catullus, Sallust, Lucan, Persius, Pliny, Varro and some other authors. He was acquainted with the letters of the Greek alphabet and the names of some Greek authors. He had a considerable knowledge of the sacred Scriptures. Some kinds of animals, of plants, of metals and of gems were known to him.

Much of his information we know to be inexact, but he was on the other hand acquainted with facts not universally known to members of universities at the present day, such as the names of the liberal arts whence masters and bachelors are designated. He had heard of MSS. written on purple vellum in gold or silver letters.

Such may have been the attainments of Cynifrid, the first physician who appears in English history and whose opinion is recorded in the first great historical work which was written in England.

Cynifrid's attainments, supposing them not to exceed what is in Isidore, seem small to us, yet the present regius professor of physic in this university is certainly the first of his office who has known the true way in which a tuberculous abscess such as that of Etheldreda is produced.

Sir Thomas Watson, a great physician, a fellow of St John's and Linacre lecturer, in the last edition of his book on medicine which received his revision and which appeared some twelve hundred years after the time of Cynifrid, calls such chronic enlargement of the glands of the neck scrofulous and inclines to the opinion that there is a scrofulous diathesis and distinct tubercular diathesis. The uniformity as to cause of all the manifestations of tubercle and the fact that the swellings and bone diseases once called scrofulous are also due to the invasion of tissues by the tubercle bacillus have only been established within living memory.

I venture to mention this because in criticizing the ignorance of the Dark Ages or the Middle Ages modern writers often forget how very ignorant we ourselves are, or how recent is our knowledge.

At the death-bed of the Conqueror we have the prognosis of the physicians but not their diagnosis.

"Consulti medici urinæ inspectione mortem citissimam prædixerunt," says William of Malmesbury who might have talked with men who knew Gilbert of Lisieux and the abbot of Jumièges, the king's physicians, *archiatri* as the chronicler calls them, reminding one of the kings of the Heptarchy who in early charters at Westminster Abbey appear as witnesses with the title Basileus.

In the summer of 1087, William the Conqueror had lost his usual activity and had lain ill in bed at Rouen. Of his symptoms we only know this languor and that he had a distended abdomen. He had long been fat, "immensæ corpulentiæ" says Malmesbury, but this was more than the "obesitas ventris" which had deformed him, for the king of France, coarsely jesting, enquired if he was lying in. The king of the English swore by the resurrection and glory of God "cum ad missam post partum iero, centum millia candelas ei libabo."

He rose from his bed, mounted his horse, and took and burned Mantes in the last week of July, according to Ordericus Vitalis. The heat of the weather and of the fire and his exertions made him worse. William of Malmesbury, who had not remembered the king's previous confinement to bed, says that these causes originated his disease. As to the familiar story of a blow from the pommel of his saddle due to his horse treading on hot ashes or jumping a ditch the historian merely gives it as a report, saying of it " Dicunt quidam." Ordericus Vitalis, a writer of the same generation as William of Malmesbury, also attributes the king's illness to his exertions and the heat of the weather and says nothing of an accident but only that the final illness lasted six weeks. It was clearly the continuation of that from which he had suffered before he started for Mantes. The account of his burial after such an illness and with the particulars mentioned by William of Jumièges suggests an obstruction of the large intestine. He was aged about sixty and the most probable cause of a partial obstruction accompanied by loss of strength for some three months was a new growth. If this were primary in the descending colon or lower, and in view of the patient being able to sit on his horse, the sigmoid flexure may be suggested; extensive secondary growths in the liver, which are of course very common in such cases, may have been present and may have been one of the causes of the abdominal distension. The king's resolute nature stirred by the scoffs of Philip might have enabled William to go into the war in spite of the serious nature of his illness.

In the Franco-German war, at a time when it seemed possible that England might be involved, I was asked to see a private soldier, the servant of a friend of mine, who had these conditions. I explained to him that he had better come into hospital. He agreed but said it must not be at once, "for in the present state of affairs I should not like to leave the regiment."

He had the same martial spirit as the Conqueror. The common bile duct is not unlikely in such a case to be partly obstructed by a mass of new growth and hence the definite appearance on which the physicians based their prognosis may have been a deep bile stain. The patient's dangerous state was doubtless sufficiently declared by his general condition when he came back to Rouen.

The way in which the Conqueror died, a gradual sinking from weakness with a mind unclouded by the rise of temperature which would have accompanied a peritonitis, is common in new growths of this kind. It is not necessary to believe that he delivered the long speeches attributed to him by William of Malmesbury and Ordericus Vitalis, but it is clear that he settled his affairs spiritual and temporal, tried to set right some of the wrong he had done and indicated the distribution of his dominions amongst his sons. The actual termination of his life is consistent with the opinion I have expressed. On Thursday, September 9, 1087, according to Ordericus, at the beginning of sunrise the king was waked by the bell of the cathedral of Rouen and asked what had rung. On hearing in the answer the words "in the church of St Mary," he raised his hands and asked her prayers for his reconciliation "with her Son, our Lord, Jesus Christ," and with these words immediately died.

I remember a patient in St Bartholomew's with a new growth of the colon who died in this way. It was obvious that her strength was rapidly failing but though very weak she had talked quite clearly the day before. The next morning, a little later than William of Normandy, she raised one arm, placed her hand upon her chest and immediately died. She had a large antemortem clot in her right ventricle and this with the ill-nourished condition of the myocardium, a part of her general wasting, caused her heart to cease to beat. Exactly such was the death of William the Conqueror.

Some of the mediæval physicians and perhaps a majority were ecclesiastics like William's *archiatri,* as for example Albert, the physician, who went with Lanfranc to see Egelward a lunatic and who afterwards became a cardinal, and John of St Giles, the friend and physician of Robert Grosseteste, bishop of Lincoln, who cured the earl of Gloucester from an attack of what was thought poisoning, and Ranulphus Besace, physician to Richard I, who told Matthew Paris about the death of the Prince of Antioch which he witnessed. What a terrible occasion it was. The Prince had been taken prisoner by Saladin and long kept in heavy chains. Ranulphus was sent to try and obtain his release. The prisoner was brought in with his arms bound and when asked by Saladin what he would do if their situations were changed said, with many insulting expressions, that he would have himself cut off Saladin's head. There was no time for Dr Ranulphus Besace to intervene, for Saladin stood up, called for his sword, and with one blow cut off the Christian captive's head.

Another ecclesiastic and physician, was Nicholas Tynchewyke, who lectured at Oxford on medicine and of whom Edward I on October 7, 1306 says

to whom, after God, we owe thanks for our recovery from the illness which lately oppressed us (Rymer, *Fœdera*, II. 1077–8)

and who held the living of Reculver.

Others like Master William le Provencall, physician to Alianora mother of Edward I, who was given leave to go abroad with her in February 1275 (Rymer II. 44), are not stated to have been in holy orders.

Books became more numerous and the authors quoted in any treatise on medicine, such as the *Compendium* of Gilbertus Anglicus, the *Rosa Anglica* of John of Gaddesden, the *Lilium Medicinæ* of Bernard of Gordon or the *Breviarium Bartholomei* of John Mirfeld, show how much reading a physician went through. It is clear that experience of patients would now and then break in and enlighten him, but his formal studies began and ended with books and learning things at the bedside was no compulsory part of his education. The history of Gilbertus Anglicus is obscure (Dr J. F. Payne was working at it shortly before his death), John of Gaddesden certainly practised in London, while John Mirfeld lived in the Augustinian Priory of St Bartholomew in Smithfield.

Though for the most part isolated so far as their profession was concerned, physicians in England throughout the Middle Ages were in contact with the learning of their time.

Their position was something like that of a medical fellow in a college here in the period when such fellowships were given to men who had studied or would study medicine.

They spent their days in conversational and social relations with men occupied with other parts of learning.

The illustrious originator of this lectureship first brought physicians together in England by the foundation in London of the College of Physicians.

The College was constituted by Letters Patent dated September 23, 1518, the tenth year of King Henry VIII.

The document is preserved in the College. It states that the king was moved to follow the example of several cities in Italy to found a College in London of learned and grave men who therein and for seven miles round should practise medicine and should prevent improper practice.

To this he was urged on the petition of six physicians and of Thomas, cardinal priest of St Cecilia in Trastavere, archbishop of York and Chancellor of England. The College was to have a perpetual succession and a common seal and was to have the power of electing a President annually and was to contain a court of four censors with judicial functions.

The grant of the letters is witnessed by Cuthbert Tonstall, then Master of the Rolls.

Linacre, who was in the true sense the founder and in whose house the College began to meet and continued its meetings for nearly a century, is mentioned second among the six physicians who petitioned for the foundation, probably because John Chambre, who had been physician to Henry VII and whose name is placed first, was his senior among the royal physicians. Chambre was physician and friend of William Warham, archbishop of Canterbury, by whom Linacre was encouraged in his translations of Galen and to whom Linacre in the evening of his life dedicated his version of Galen's *De Naturalibus Facultatibus*, anxious to show his gratitude to the archbishop "ubi per morbi sævitiam liceret," for the physician was then ill and in frequent pain. Warham died eight years after Linacre. The account which Erasmus gives of his death in his introduction to the 1534 edition of St Jerome's works shows Warham's nature and what an honour it was to be admitted to his friendship. His treasury was nearly empty owing to his wise and generous expenditure for his see and for the advancement of learning. "Moreover, it being made known to him by his household that there were hardly thirty gold pieces of money left in his chest, he said joyfully : it is well : I always longed to die thus : it is enough of travelling money for me soon hence to depart."

A like contempt for the accumulation of wealth was part of the character which Linacre desired to impress on the physicians of his college.

Linacre and Francis, the fifth of the six physicians mentioned in the Letters Patent, were both frequenters of Wolsey's house.

"Oh grand and happy house," says Erasmus, "oh truly magnificent cardinal, who has such men as his councillors, whose table is surrounded by such luminaries."

Wolsey's influence was no doubt of service to Linacre in obtaining the Letters Patent.

The cardinal is remembered in a much less degree in relation to medicine at St Bartholomew's Hospital, where the chapter of the hospital appointed him on two occasions to nominate a master. In 1525 he was preparing for the endowment of his colleges at Oxford and at Ipswich and nominated Alexander Colyns, prior of Daventry, the estates of which were to be used for these colleges, to the mastership of St Bartholomew's. Colyns died in 1528 and Wolsey nominated Edward Staple, afterwards bishop of Meath, who held office till 1532, and is perhaps now best remembered as the man who urged Henry VIII to assume the title which except an occasional use by pretenders had fallen into disuse since the death of Maelsheachlainn MacDomhnaill, Rex Hiberniæ, in 1022. "I pray God," says Linacre, in his dedication of Galen's *De pulsuum usu* to Wolsey, "that you may be well and live for many happy years the distinguished Mæcenas of letters."

The seventeen fellows of the College of

Physicians then living would all think of the terrific storm of St Andrew's Eve 1530 as marking in their memories the unhappy end of the cardinal who had supported their founder's intentions and was always to be remembered as a benefactor, and what they knew of him was best expressed in the lines

> He was a scholar, and a ripe and good one ;
> Exceeding wise, fair spoken and persuading.

Erasmus has shown his admiration of Linacre as a scholar and as a physician in many passages, as in his well-known letter to Paulus Bombasius of July 26, 1518, "Thomas Linacre is the physician of the court, it would be waste of time to dwell upon this man to you since what he is he himself demonstrates in his published books," and in that to Richard Pace in October 1518, "At length Galen translated by Linacre begins to appear in the bookshops, a work that pleases me beyond measure," and in that to

Ægidius Bushidius, " I send as a gift the books of Galen, the work of Thomas Linacre, now speaking better in Latin than they erstwhile spoke in Greek."

He shows too that he appreciated Linacre's medical advice. After a journey to Paris, Erasmus had a severe headache and swollen glands in his neck, throbbing temples, buzzing in both ears "and all the time there is no Linacre at hand who might free me by his art," and in another letter, " I beg you to send me written out the remedy which, when I was last in London, I took on your recommendation, for the boy left the prescription at the apothecary's. It will be a great kindness to me. The rest of my news you will know from More. Farewell. From St Omers, June 5, 1506."

Dr Francis, the fifth of the physicians in the Letters Patent, is mentioned by Erasmus as a well tried friend.

Erasmus pronounced an oration[1],

In laudem artis medicæ,

addressed to graduates and students of medicine[2], which he revised some years later and sent to Asinius Lyranus, a distinguished physician, on March 13, 1518. He treats the subject chiefly as a student of antiquity, a classical scholar and a theologian, but also points out the variety contained in the study and its worthiness to be the occupation of a life-time.

The oration exhibits the friendly feeling of Erasmus towards medicine, a feeling shown also in other passages of his writings.

As in the letter which he wrote for a friend who wished to make a present of a Greek Homer, not improbably the beautiful Florentine

---

[1] *Encomia Medicinæ* : Rotterdam, 1644.

[2] " Vobis igitur magnopere gratulor, eximii viri, quibus contigit in hoc pulcherrimo genere professionis excellere : Vos adhortor, optimi iuvenes, hanc toto pectore complectimini," p. 105.

editio princeps of 1488, to his physician, and in
that to a student of medicine in Paris,

"Since you long for our Aphorisms beware
lest you imagine them of the same kind as those
of your Hippocrates. The subject is different,
but if you ask for a little book of Erasmus 'De
institutione principis Christiani' by the title you
will soon find it. Farewell : Antwerp 1516."

Thus the phrases of his declamation were not
merely pieces of rhetoric used for a particular
occasion but represent his constant frame of
mind. Erasmus was the friend of the founder,
and of the College of Physicians itself and of
its subjects of study. Nothing could more
clearly show what was the intellectual position
of physicians in England at the Renaissance.
That Archbishop Warham, Cuthbert Tonstall
and Sir Thomas More were his friends tells
much of Linacre's character and learning. His
works complete our view of him. They show

his desire to make Galen known in his time and the encouragement of scholarship for its own sake and of Greek as the guide to the true sources of medicine and of the careful study of Latin as the means of addressing the learned world.

Since the figure which the physician makes in English history in addition to his own increase of knowledge is as the associate and friend of other learned men, and that it is in these ways that he has exercised most influence on his time since the foundation of the College of Physicians, it is worth observing how the founder was associated with two great men in the other two faculties.

Tonstall, More, Linacre—these three great Englishmen represent the three great faculties and each shows by his writings as well outside as within his faculty that wakefulness of mind which adds so much to usefulness in a profession and in life.

Tonstall received the latter part of his education at Cambridge and knew Greek so well that Erasmus says in a letter to William Latimer, the classical scholar:

" To say exactly what I feel, if it happened that I had Linacre or Tonstall for a teacher I should not long for Italy."

Tonstall had a busy career. Archbishop Warham made him rector of Harrow. In 1515 he was sent ambassador to Brussels to Charles, Prince of Castile. In May 1516 he became Master of the Rolls, in 1519 ambassador to Charles V at Cologne, in 1521 dean of Salisbury and in 1522 bishop of London. In May 1523 he was keeper of the Privy Seal, in 1525 ambassador to Charles V at Toledo and in 1527 ambassador to France. In 1530 he became bishop of Durham and in 1537 President of the North. In 1551 he wrote his book *De Veritate corporis et sanguinis Domini Nostri*

Jesu Christi in Eucharistia. Outside these responsible offices Tonstall was mixed up in a vast amount of public business and that he took a solemn view of his responsibilities as a divine is shown in many ways, as in his pleasant dedication of his treatise on arithmetic *De Arte supputandi* in 1522 to More.

Tonstall therein explains that the money transactions of public business made him again go over arithmetic and think upon it, and read all the writings he could find about it whether learned or unlearned, Latin or vernacular. Then he had thought out the difficulties of the subject and arranged and improved his explanations, following the example of a bear licking its unformed cubs into shape. "He had just," he says (this was in 1522), "been appointed to the bishopric of London and must give the rest of his life to sacred literature and throw aside profane writings, and first of all these commentaries on the art of calculation." He did not like to burn the result of the studies of so many nights and so sent the book to press.

More attained the chief place in his profession and his *Utopia* belongs to the permanent literature of civilized nations. He was the delight of the learned of his time and his goodness was felt by all his contemporaries. His steadfastness in his principles when that firmness brought him loss of station, property and life is one of the greatest and most splendid examples in history. Though in *Utopia* jewels were only the ornaments of children, yet in figuring his career I must compare his death to a single great diamond in a crown ornamented with many jewels but in which the refulgence of this one gem draws away our gaze from the great brightness of many of the others. His Greek, his minute knowledge of English, his

imagination, his wit, his conduct in all relations
and parts of life put him above all other sages
of the law in England as the most shining
example of their profession. This is the conclusion of our time : in his own, before the whole
splendour of his character had appeared, Erasmus
thought him one "whose incomparable charm
is due not only to the Muses and the Graces
but also to his wit."

Such were the divine and the lawyer. The
physician was worthy of their company. Linacre
has rendered incalculable service to medicine
in England by his devotion to learning and
determination by means of learning to improve
his profession or rather to establish its followers
as a profession bound together for the increase
of knowledge and in the service of the public,
which they were not before. His influence is
felt to this day.

MORE was for all time a noble example.

Tonstall accomplished the arduous and complicated work which fell to his share in his own day. What Linacre did was of service to his own time and has continued to be useful to many succeeding generations.

It was not merely what he had seen of colleges in Italy which made Linacre anxious to found one in London. It was his observation of the good effect of continued association with the learned.

Linacre knew this and founded a college in which by constant association physicians might continually be improved in learning, in the practice and in the morals of their profession. Such was the College of Physicians of London.

He was its first president. His ideas were confirmed and continued by John Caius, who some thirty years later succeeded him as president.

There is so noble a memorial of him here

and Dr Venn has so fully and so admirably elucidated his life and his works, that it would be presumptuous in me to add to that well drawn and well deserved panegyric. Yet Caius, besides being a continuator of Linacre, shows in his life another aspect of the physician in English history, that of a founder and improver of the means of learning.

The college with beautiful gates with which Caius ornamented Cambridge and the great dome of the Radcliffe library, the Infirmary and the Observatory at Oxford, and Radcliffe's benefactions there, show that physicians have taken a share in increasing the means of attaining knowledge in the ancient universities, and even a greater effect has been produced by Sir Hans Sloane, who like Linacre and Caius was president of the College of Physicians, for his bequest to the nation was the origin of the British Museum.

The effect of Linacre's College has been great in producing and maintaining a society of learned physicians acquainted with one another and in constant touch with the world of learning.

The Royal Society, so effectual in its promotion of science, may justly be regarded as an offshoot from Linacre's, since it arose from the conversational meeting of a dozen learned men of whom a third were physicians round the table of Wilkins at Wadham College and the success of these has indirectly or directly led to all the other learned societies of England.

It was just a hundred years after Linacre translated Proclus on the Sphere that Dr William Gilbert, one of the many ornaments of St John's, published his treatise on the Magnetism of the Earth. Harvey's lectures containing the doctrine of the Circulation came next and then his book in 1628 and then Glisson's *De Rachitide*, the first regular pathological treatise in England.

Thus had the study of the Greek observers, of Hippocrates and of Galen, led not to antiquarianism but to original observation and discovery.

The physician who had taken a large share in the revival of Greek learning which so mightily affected the studies and thoughts of the nation now led the way into the paths of science.

The College itself early in its career had established a botanic garden and made Gerard, the surgeon and writer of the Herbal, its superintendent.

Nor were these advances only in the Natural Sciences, for Sir William Petty may justly be regarded as one of the founders of statistical studies and Political Economy in England.

Thomas Lodge is the earliest Doctor of Physic—he graduated at Avignon and became a Licentiate of the College of Physicians in

1610—whose writings deserve to be regarded as important contributions to English literature.

Cowley had taken a medical degree and Locke did so at the age of forty-two, but neither of the poets nor the philosopher ever belonged in any full sense to the world of medicine, though Lodge had some practice and Locke did what he could for the precarious health of Shaftesbury

> A fiery soul, which working out its way,
> Fretted the pigmy body to decay
> And o'erinformed the tenement of clay,

and not infrequently turned his mind to medical questions as is shown by his letters.

It is not till the end of the seventeenth century and beginning of the eighteenth that regular physicians begin to appear in the literature of England, Garth first and then Arbuthnot. That the physician did not appear earlier in this field was because his language of expression, he being pre-eminently a citizen of the world, was generally Latin.

'The Dispensary' of Garth is a poem on a medical subject interesting for half a century, while the controversy of which it treats was known to the public, always a respectable example of English verse and containing some lines preserved in general memory.

'The Dispensary' has for its frontispiece the Theatrum Cutlerianum built by Sir John Cutler, one of the fellows, for the College of Physicians in Warwick Lane of which a wooden model is preserved in the present College in Pall Mall East. The theatre is entered by a classical portal above which rises a hexagonal building with a domed roof terminated by a short spire surmounted by a golden ball.

> There stands a Dome, Majestick to the Sight,
> And sumptuous arches bear its oval height;
> A golden Globe placed high with artful skill,
> Seems to the distant Sight a gilded Pill.
> This Pile was, by the Pious Patrons Aim,
> Rais'd for a use as noble as its frame;

> Nor did the learn'd Society decline
> The Propagation of that great Design.
> In all her Mazes, Nature's Face they viewed,
> And as she disappeared, they still pursued.

Such is the poet's description of the College and of its building.

The subject of his poem was a feud within the College and with the apothecaries as to the establishment of a Dispensary for the Sick Poor, and its object was to put an end to the warfare. The poem begins with the plots and incantations of the apothecaries, and gives descriptions of the physicians on each side, such as that of Dr Edward Tyson :

> When for advice the Vulgar throng, he's found
> With lumber of vile books besieged around ;
> The gazing fry acknowledge their surprize,
> Consulting less their Reason than their Eyes.
> And he perceives it stands in greater stead,
> To furnish well his Classes, than his Head.
> Thus a weak State, by wise Distrust, enclines
> To num'rous Stores, and strength in Magazines.
> So Fools are always most profuse of Words
> And Cowards never fail of longest Swords.

Abandoned Authors here a refuge meet,
And from the world to dust and worms retreat;
Here Dregs and Sediments of auctions reign,
Refuse of fairs and gleanings of Duck Lane,
And up these shelves much Gothic lumber climbs
With Swiss philosophy and Danish Rhimes.

The author follows well his own precept

Harsh words, though pertinent, uncouth appear,
None please the fancy, who offend the Ear.
Read Wycherley, consider Dryden well,
In one what rigorous turns of fancy shine
In th' other, *Syrens* warble in each line.

In the fifth of the six cantos of the poem a battle between the contending parties is described, and in the sixth Harvey is sought in the Elysian fields, and deploring that the controversy interferes with useful researches advises that Somers, " the matchless Atticus," acting as a visitor should settle the quarrel.

Steele in his dedication of ' The Lover and Reader' says that an epistle directed ' To the Best-natur'd Man ' would find its way to Garth without his name.

This kindly feeling is shown in the most poetic lines of the poem, which did not appear till the fifth or sixth edition

> 'Tis to the Vulgar, Death too harsh appears ;
> The ill we feel is only in our Fears.
> To Die, is Landing on some silent shoar,
> Where Billows never break, nor Tempests roar :
> E'er well we feel the friendly Stroke, 'tis o'er.
> The Wise through Thought th' Insults of Death defy ;
> The Fools, through blessed Insensibility.
> 'Tis what the Guilty fear, the Pious crave ;
> Sought by the Wretch, and vanquish'd by the Brave.
> It eases Lovers, sets the Captive free ;
> And, tho' a Tyrant, offers Liberty.

The man who had it in him to write these lines deserved the honour which came to him of providing ceremonial and respect for the body of Dryden, who died poor and neglected. Garth obtained leave to bring the great poet's remains to the College of Physicians whence they were conveyed to Westminster Abbey. The printed ticket, which was probably the composition of Garth, is

Sir, You are desired to Accompany the corps of Mr John Dryden, from the College of Physicians in Warwick Lane, to Westminster Abby ; on Monday the 13th of this Instant May, 1700. At Four of the Clock in the Afternoon exactly, it being resolved to be moving by Five a Clock And be pleased to bring this Ticket with you.

Pope wrote the prologue, Garth the epilogue of Addison's 'Cato.' The more famous poet in sententious lines prepares the audience for the serious drama they are to see, but Garth feels that everyone has had enough of gloom and tragedy. Marcia, the daughter of Cato, had been beloved by both Juba and Sempronius, and Garth at once relieves the dulness by making Mrs Porter, the actress who spoke the Epilogue, burst into a laughing argument on the subject first of

What odd fantastick Things we Women do !
Who wou'd not listen when young Lovers woo ?

and then of the worldly prudence of modern times, ending with a regret for the past

Oh ! may once more the happy age appear
When Words were artless and the Thoughts sincere.

This pointed, airy way of speaking was characteristic of Garth. Arbuthnot with a few touches depicts his manner in 'The History of John Bull.' There is to be a consultation on John Bull's mother:

"Physicians were sent for in haste: Sir Roger, with great difficulty, brought Radcliffe; Garth came upon the first message. There were several others called in but, as usual upon such occasions, they differed strangely at the consultation. At last they divided into two parties, one sided with Garth, the other with Radcliffe. *Dr Garth*. 'This case seems to me to be plainly hysterical; the old woman is whimsical; it is a common thing for your old women to be so; I'll pawn my life, blisters with the steel diet, will recover her.'"

Garth in his epilogue had appeared in literary association with Addison. His regard for Somers is shown in the couplet

Somers does sickening Equity restore
And helpless orphans are oppress't no more

and in the last canto of ' The Dispensary.'

Somers is most often spoken of as a great lawyer and pillar of the constitution, the composer of the Bill of Rights, one of the patriarchs of Whig principles as established at the Revolution, but here and there glimpses of him appear which show that his literary and historical con‧ versation were delightful. To mention but one, Thomas Madox, the historian of the Exchequer, a man full of learning and incapable of servility or adulation :

" Amongst the Patrons it (the science of antiquities) hath in the present age, Your Lordship may justly be placed in the upper rank. But in regard the other Bodies of Learned men in the Civil Community may affirm each for themselves, that You are a Master of Their Science ; the Antiquaries must

be content to have such share in Your Lordship, as is consistent with the Just Claim of the
Learned of other Faculties."

The famous Kit Cat Club, to which Garth
and Somers and Addison, Dorset and Prior
belonged, brought the physician into close relation with the literature of his time. In it
his influence was felt and as the members ate
mutton pies and too often sent round the wine
some of the best talk of the age went on.

Not indeed all, for another fellow of the
College of Physicians lived in the intimacy of a
different society. The circumferences of these
two circles touched though those members
who were active politicians belonged to hostile
parties. At this other table sat Swift and Pope
and Arbuthnot ; and Harley, Bolingbroke and
Gay were at times allowed seats which in the
presence of these three they did not deserve.
And of the three Swift was the most powerful,

a man unlike any other in English history and whose life and writings will always affect both the mind and the feelings of everyone who tries to become acquainted with him. He had arrived at a conclusion, unaffected, horrible but to him irresistible, to hate mankind not out of mere inhumanity or self-conceit on his part but as a result of long observation, a conclusion that made him wretched till he reached the place

ubi sæva indignatio
ulterius cor lacerare nequit.

He yet said

" Oh! if the world had but a dozen Arbuthnots in it I would burn my travels."

Physicians who have great opportunities of observing them have generally felt kindly towards their species and Arbuthnot shone in this opinion. Pope was not quite worthy of the other two for he was dominated by a love of himself and a covetousness of fame from which they were free.

His conduct as regards the publication of his own letters, his intrigues with Orrery as to Swift's correspondence show him to have been a less man than Swift or Arbuthnot, and his life was so full of untruthfulness that the most learned of his editors, tired of detecting his crafts and frauds during many years, one day sent for a cart and having packed his papers and pamphlets into boxes placed them thereon and sent them away determined to have no more to do with such a man.

In the actual presence of Swift, Pope was afraid not to be truthful and in that of Arbuthnot felt disinclined to be anything else, so that his best qualities and his real love of literature came out in their presence and therefore both cared for him though it is easy to discover that both had seen through him.

When Swift speaking of his own death said

> Poor Pope will grieve a month and Gay
> A week: and Arbuthnot a day,

he was not attributing heartlessness to his friend but was thinking of him as "the most cheerful creature that ever breathed[1]."

None but Arbuthnot could have written without fear to Swift

"I have as good a right to invade your solitude as Lord Bolingbroke, Gay, or Pope, and you see I make use of it. I know you wish us all at the devil for robbing a moment from your vapours and vertigo. It is no matter for that; you shall have a sheet of paper every post till you come to yourself. By a paragraph in yours to Mr Pope, I find you are in the case of the man who held the whole night by a broom-bush and found when daylight appeared he was within two inches of the ground. You

---

[1] Lewis to Swift, June 30, 1737.

don't seem to know how well you stand with our great folks. I myself have been at a great man's table, and have heard, out of the mouths of violent Irish Whigs, the whole table talk turn upon your commendation. If it had not been on the general topic of your good qualities, and the good you did, I should have grown jealous of you. My intention in this is not to expostulate, but to do you good. I know how unhappy a vertigo makes anybody, that has the misfortune to be troubled with it. I might have been deep in it myself, if I had a mind, and will propose a cure for you, that I will pawn my reputation upon. I have of late sent several patients in that case to the Spa, to drink there of the Geronster water, which will not carry from the spot. It has succeeded marvellously with them all."

Arbuthnot's *History of John Bull* has established that name in English parlance and like all his prose is both vigorous and clear.

The original draft of his poem Γνῶθι Σεαυτὸν in his own hand is in the British Museum. Most readers will think that only some of his alterations were for the better but in either form it is an admirable poem and its commencement noble:

> What am I? how produced? and for what end?
> Whence drew I being? to what period tend?
> Am I th' abandoned orphan of blind chance,
> Dropt by wild atoms in disordered dance?
> Or from an endless chain of causes wrought?
> And of unthinking substance Born with thought.
> The purple stream, that through my vessels glides,
> Dull and unconscious Flows like common tides.
> The pipes through which the circling juices stray
> Are not that thinking I, no more than they.
> This Frame compacted with transcendent skill
> Of moving joynts obedient to my will,
> Nurs'd from the fruitfull Glebe, like yonder Tree,
> Waxes and wastes, 'tis mine but 'tis not me.
> New matter still my mouldering Mass sustains
> The Fabrick chang'd, the Tenant still remains.

It is a testimony to the power of Arbuthnot's

mind that he was untouched by the misanthropy of Swift and though in frequent contact with the intriguing Pope was always truthful and straightforward. I dwell upon these merits because they show what the influence of this physician was on these geniuses of his time. Indeed Swift's remark on the dozen Arbuthnot's shows this clearly and it appears in several of Pope's letters.

Great as was the conversation of the beginning of the eighteenth century, much as we could wish for evenings with the Kit Cat Club or with Pope, Swift, and Arbuthnot, the greatest of all recorded English conversation is that of the latter half of the same century. Interest in it has never flagged since the incomparable Boswell laid his record of it before the world. It was chiefly conversation of men who cared for books and life, and while every reading man studies it, it seems to have an especial charm for men of letters. Croker tried to increase the store, a man not devoid of literary perception though belonging to an age when the precision of science was rarely applied to literature and when English libraries contained, with the exception of Gibbon and Hallam, few exact historical books except the ponderous tomes of Dugdale, and Le Neve, and Rymer, and Newcourt and Madox and Tanner, vast store-houses of knowledge which no man could read who ran, but only he who would sit before a lectern for months. Macaulay threw some light on the record in his severe exposure of Croker's errors. Whitwell Elwin, perhaps the only man of the reign of Queen Victoria who if he had lived in London would at once have been like Johnson the centre of a great literary circle and the delight of every person, literary or not literary, young or old, with whom he talked, left a wonderful picture of the moral and literary splendour of Johnson and Burke. Leslie Stephen, exact, concise, full of literature and of human feeling, added his picture from a different standpoint. Birkbeck Hill appeared as the Gronovius of Johnson and left no passage unexplained and no name unindexed. Raleigh, a glory of this university though writing in another, has shown his just confidence in his own powers and insight into literature by his six Johnsonian essays, and John Bailey in this year, rightly undeterred by all that had been written before, has produced a book fresh and original throughout, showing, more fully and clearly than had been shown before, Johnson's relation to the habits of thought and the sentiments of the English nation, how great an Englishman he was and ever will be.

Thus from their own time to ours have the thoughts and words of the Johnsonian circle influenced the nation. In this great company

of Johnson and Burke and Goldsmith and
Reynolds, Dr Richard Brocklesby was also a
figure well able both to take part in the conversation and to enjoy it. He was a senior
boy at Ballitore school when Burke went there
on May 26, 1741, and the friendship thus begun
lasted their lives. It is interesting to trace a
slight resemblance in their handwriting due no
doubt to both having been well taught in that
famous school on the banks of the river Griese.
Brocklesby's *Œconomical and Medical Obser-
vations from* 1758 *to* 1763 was the first attempt
to state the necessary conditions for the pre-
servation of health in barrack and camp life.
He was incorporated M.D. at Cambridge in
1754 and elected a fellow of the College of
Physicians in 1756. Besides being excellent
in his profession and full of many kinds of
learning he was like Garth and Arbuthnot a
model of generosity. He gave Burke when in

need of money a thousand pounds and wrote that he would gladly repeat the gift every year. He offered Johnson when he was thinking of going to Italy a hundred a year for life. He attended him often and in his last illness.

The account of one of his last visits to Johnson illustrates well their relations of friendship and of literature :

"About eight or ten days before his death, when Dr Brocklesby paid him his morning visit, he seemed very low and desponding, and said 'I have been as a dying man all night.' He then emphatically broke out in the words of Shakespeare,

> Canst thou not minister to a mind diseased,
> Pluck from the memory a rooted sorrow ;
> Raze out the written troubles of the brain
> And, with some sweet oblivious antidote,
> Cleanse the stuff'd bosom of that perilous stuff,
> Which weighs upon the heart.

to which Dr Brocklesby readily answered from the same great poet :

> Therein the patient
> Must minister to himself.

Johnson expressed himself much satisfied with the application."

Such were the relations of Brocklesby to Burke and to Johnson.

I chose as the title of this lecture " The Physician in English History." I wished to discuss the question of what effect he has had on the nation besides that of his scientific discoveries, and of their application to his practice.

Those men deserve to be remembered in history who have added to the happiness of mankind : who have lengthened and gladdened life, to use Johnson's words : who have enlarged and opened men's minds.

These merits physicians in England may claim. They took a large share in the establishment of Greek learning, which was the first step to modern science.

They have made additions not only to their own science but to every science relating to it. They with their colleagues the surgeons originated the regular service of hospitals and have always freely given their time and their skill to it. They have built up with the surgeons medical education in England with scarcely any help from the revenues or powers of the state. They have always set an active example of compassion for the poor, the sick and the injured. These things are important in the history of a nation. It would be easy to give a whole course of lectures on what physicians have done in these ways, but in this single Linacre lecture I have tried no more than to indicate the position of physicians in the conversation and thought of their time and their influence on the genius of each generation.

Milton Keynes UK
Ingram Content Group UK Ltd.
UKHW041519181024
449640UK00009B/75